The Doctor's Guide to:

Life threatening Allergic reactions

ANAPHYLAXIS

Caused by Food allergies or insect stings

by Kenneth Wright

In consultation with Dr. Philip Lieberman and adapted from the notes and articles, with permission from: Dr. Barry Zimmerman, Dr. H.A. Sampson, Dr. Mendelson, Dr. K.G. Sweeney, Dr. G. Settipane and Dr. J.H. Barnard.

Our thanks for the use of patient education material from the American Academy of Allergy Asthma & Immunology Allergy Asthma , The American College of Asthma and Immunology, The American Academy of Pediatrics, the Allergy / Asthma Information Association and the Medic Alert Foundation.

Disclaimer: the content of this brochure is for informational purposes only. It is not intended to replace evaluation by a physician.

For more information and to see our full catalogue, visit www.mediscript.net or email: mediscript30@yahoo.ca

Printed in USA

1SBN 978-1550407884

FORWARD

There is one theme that runs through the practice of medicine, regardless of one's specialty or the disease being treated: this theme is that knowledge empowers the patient.

Patients who are equipped with knowledge can favorably affect the outcome of their condition, and deal with it in a much more effective manner. Unfortunately, the converse is also true – the patient not equipped with knowledge does not, as a rule, far as well.

Perhaps there is no other condition so profoundly affected by the presence or absence of this knowledge as anaphylaxis. This explosive, unpredictable and potentially fatal reaction does not allow time to ponder. In order to manage it adequately, the patient requires knowledge of both prevention and therapy in the case of an acute event. The therapy must be swift and instinctive in order to be truly effective. One can only put this therapy into action of he or she has knowledge about the condition.

I possibly feel more strongly about this issue than many other physicians because of my own personal experience with anaphylactic episodes. I have been fortunate enough to have had the opportunity of learning from patients over a 30-year time span; the one thing I've learned is that the better we teach, and the greater knowledge on the part of the patient, the better the results. It has taken a number of years to refine this teaching process to the point where I have been able to considerably reduce morbidity and therefore enhance our patients' quality of life.

Over the past 30-plus years, I have had the opportunity to review numerous education aids written for patients who experience anaphylactic events

– this little manual is certainly one of the best. It is well-organized, quite easy to read, and immensely instructive. It not only serves to emphasize the major features of education regarding anaphylactic episodes, but also points patients to resources that are available for further educational opportunities.

Unless one has personally experienced an episode of anaphylaxis, or has a relative – especially a child – who has been through such an event, one cannot appreciate the effect on the quality of life and the burden exerted by this condition. Living in fear of a repeat reaction, or fearing that your child will have such an event, profoundly alters ones activities and outlook. Tools such as this effective advice manual reduce the impact of anaphylaxis by educating patients in the proper preventive and treatment techniques, thus supplying them with a degree of confidence and allaying fears of the unknown.

I would suggest, therefore, that anyone at risk of experiencing an episode of anaphylaxis possess this text.

Dr. Philip Lieberman

How to use this book

This book has two objectives, one to provide basic information to help a person (adult or child) prevent an anaphylactic attack. Secondly, information is provided on how to treat an anaphylaxis reaction.

The reader could be a parent or caregiver for a child or teenager at risk for anaphylaxis or you could be an adult who has developed a risk for an anaphylaxis attack.

The information should be useful to both types of readers and you take out the information most relevant for yourself.

The table of contents pinpoints the "stand alone" topics which you can reference when necessary.

It is important to note that every person at risk for anaphylaxis is unique with regard to a host of factors such as the daily activities situation, what you are allergic to, the onset of symptoms, whether asthma is also present, whether the child takes a school bus etc , there are a lot of variables.

With this complexity factor in mind we suggest you assimilate the information as a platform for comprehensively understanding anaphylaxis. However we strongly advocate you always seek definitive advice from your health care provider.

Most health care professionals highly recommend this basic information is understood by people caring for someone who is at risk to anaphylaxis or indeed if you are an adult who is at risk. It is absolutely critical for a caregiver of a patient to know exactly what to do in case of an emergency situation of anaphylaxis.

For the most part the tips suggested in the book are well accepted non controversial common sense approaches. Websites are listed to provide further research contacts.

TABLE OF CONTENTS

Introduction

"Severe Allergic Reaction, "life threatening allergy" – sounds a little scary, right? However dramatic you may think the title of this book is, it's not just meant to frighten you. It's a way of getting your attention focused on a health risk issue that is actually life threatening in a short period of time (minutes sometimes) for you or your child.

Essentially, anaphylaxis (pronounce an-uh-fuh-LAK-sis) is usually brought on by a food allergy (often peanuts) and insect stings or bites. There are other causes, too, such as medications, latex (balloons, elastic, kitchen cleaning gloves, adhesive bandages, condoms, elastic bands), and sometimes even exercise.

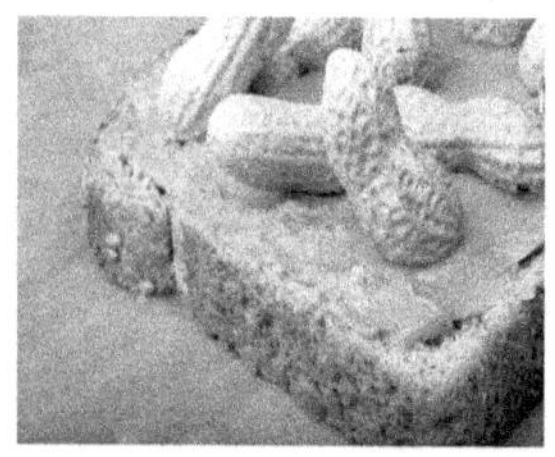

Nine groups of foods have been identified as being the most likely cause of severe allergic reaction (anaphylaxis) and account for 90% of all food anaphylactic reactions. These foods are peanuts, tree nuts (almond, Brazil nut, cashew, macadamia, hazelnut or filbert, pecan, pine nut, pistachio, walnut), cow's milk, eggs, fish, shellfish, soy, wheat and sesame seeds.

In North America there are believed to be over 200 deaths each year due food induced anaphylaxis and well over 30,000 emergency room visits. It is possible that the number of deaths may be greater due to the cause of death being listed as cardiac arrest or asthma attack, both of which can be involved with the anaphylaxis.

The statistics are disturbing: almost 13 million North Americans have food allergies, which is about 4% of the population. The incidence is higher in young children under 3 years old – one in

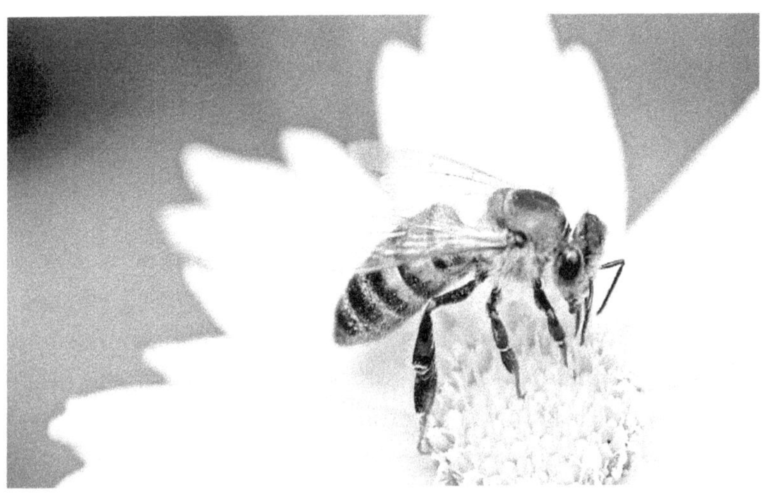

17. About 2.5 million school children have food allergies, and there is no known cure for food allergies.

The insects causing anaphylaxis are usually the stinging and biting variety like bees, yellow jackets, hornets, wasps and fire ants (which are only found in the southeastern US). These insects cause up to 150 deaths in North America each year and hundreds of thousands of hospital visits. It is believed that more than 2 million North Americans are allergic to stinging insects

Although technically an "allergy", anaphylaxis is not at all like your regular runny nose allergy where you take an antihistamine pill for gentle relief. Anaphylaxis can affect all parts of your body and sometimes can kill you in a short period of time.

The good news is that with careful planning, vigilance and communication you can almost certainly prevent an attack. By informing your place of work or school, and involving parents, caregivers, nannies, caregivers and friends, you can create a supportive and somewhat risk-free environment and enjoy a good quality of life.

The bad news is that when you have an anaphylaxis attack you cannot make an appointment with your allergist or physician for an appointment in a week's time to get medication or treatment. You have to act fast by treating yourself and calling for emergency medical help. This is a MUST.

Your physician or health care provider is always your partner in this health issue; he or she can do so much in helping you cope with the condition. But you need to take responsibility for your own survival during an anaphylaxis episode, following your health care provider's instructions and carrying out the training you have learned in order to relieve the situation.

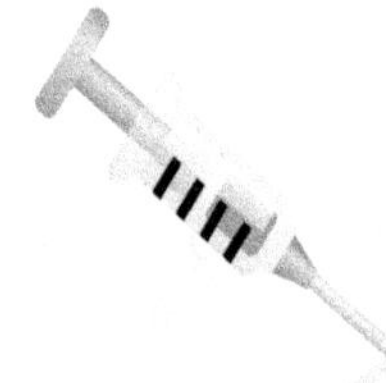

The key to saving your life or that of your child is a simple, easy to use injection of a chemical called epinephrine. If you are at risk, you or your child should always carry this auto - injector unit around with you.

This may sound simple but the prevention and treatment of anaphylaxis can be complex – not so much medically but from communication, political and environmental standpoints. The "at risk" child or adult is in danger of accidental exposure to commonly used foods and an outside environment that harbors potentially allergenic insects.

It is essential, then, to communicate the details of your allergy or that of your child with school officials, restaurant workers, airline officials, and so on. You cannot "let your guard down" for a moment because a moment is all it takes.

WHAT IS ANAPHYLAXIS

Anaphylaxis (also known as "anaphylactic shock", "allergic shock" or "severe allergic reaction") is a potentially fatal, allergic reaction. It can affect all parts of the body.

The condition usually appears in early childhood, but can develop at any age.

It must always be treated as a medical emergency, requiring immediate treatment and urgent medical attention. Anaphylaxis can involve breathing, the cardiovascular (heart and circulation) system, the skin and the gastrointestinal (digestive) tract.

Anaphylaxis occurs when a person's immune system reacts to the presence in the body of a usually harmless substance such as a food or chemicals from an insect bite resulting in an extreme body reaction.

In this case, the body's immune system is over-reacting in response to what it sees as a foreign invader or allergen entering the bloodstream. This provokes the release of massive amounts of histamine and other chemicals.

The blood vessels widen, which leads to a sudden severe lowering of blood pressure and constriction of the airways in the lungs. The reaction can begin within minutes but sometimes the reaction can occur hours after exposure to the offending agent.

The onset of anaphylaxis can be deceptive – it may be signaled by severe, but non life-threatening reactions. They can, however, become increasingly dangerous very quickly with or without subsequent exposure to the allergen. The time frame from the onset of the first symptoms to death can be as little as a few minutes if the reaction is not treated.

Further, even if symptoms subside after initial treatment, they can return as much as eight hours after exposure. It is also important to know that symptoms do not always occur in the same order, even in the same individuals.

A further "curve ball" to this condition, especially with teenagers, is that sometimes anaphylaxis can be confused with asthma, because in each case the person has difficulty breathing. Experts also believe that it is possible to have both an asthma attack and anaphylaxis at the same time. Asthma attacks, as well, can be fatal.

At this point it is good to know that an easy to use self administered injection of epinephrine (brand names of EpiPen® and Twinject®) can reverse the symptoms and possibly save your life. Your physician or pharmacist can explain and train you on usage.

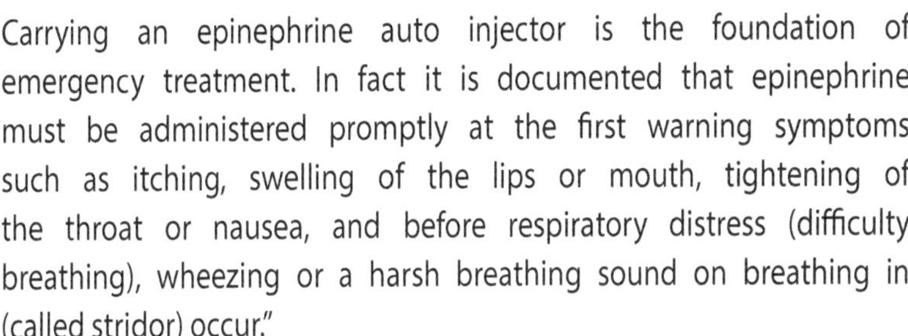

Carrying an epinephrine auto injector is the foundation of emergency treatment. In fact it is documented that epinephrine must be administered promptly at the first warning symptoms such as itching, swelling of the lips or mouth, tightening of the throat or nausea, and before respiratory distress (difficulty breathing), wheezing or a harsh breathing sound on breathing in (called stridor) occur."

Epinephrine, also known as adrenaline, is a natural hormone that the body produces in response to stress.

When you are exposed to physical stress, for example, the body kicks in with extra levels of epinephrine or adrenaline to enable you to perform better physically. These changes include relaxing the chest muscles so that you can breathe better and constricting the blood vessels to allow more blood flow to key areas of your body.

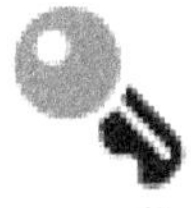

KEY FACTS

Anaphylaxis is a severe allergic reaction and CAN be life threatening. It must always be treated as a medical emergency (calling 911).

People at risk of anaphylaxis should always carry a self injection of epinephrine and immediately inject themselves during an anaphylactic reaction. The brand names are Epi Pen® or Twinject®.

RECOGNIZING ANAPHYLACTIC SYMPTOMS

Initially, these symptoms may appear mild or moderate but they can progress rapidly. The most dangerous of these reactions involve the respiratory symptom (breathing) and/or the cardiovascular system (heart and blood pressure).

It is very important to appreciate that each person at risk for an anaphylactic reaction is an individual and the timing and mix of symptoms is unique to each individual.

Not all symptoms of anaphylaxis need be present when having an attack. Symptoms do not appear in a particular order and can occur on as little as 5 minutes or several hours after exposure to the allergen be it food or an insect bite. Worse still, the life threatening reaction may progress over hours. This emphasizes the fact that no matter what the nature of the reaction is, you must seek medical help immediately.

The following page lists the common symptoms linked to the various body areas. Most symptoms are self explanatory however hives/welts are red, raised areas of the skin that itch. Stridor is the name given to a high pitched breathing sound.

Skin:	❑ Tingling of the mouth
	❑ Hives/welts (can be entirely absent, especially in severe or near-fatal cases)
	❑ Itching, or body redness
	❑ Change of skin color
	❑ Swelling of the face, lips or eyes
	❑ Red, watery eyes, runny nose
	❑ Tingling or warm sensations
	❑ Pale and floppy (young children)
Gastro - intestinal (Digestive):	❑ Difficulty swallowing
	❑ Vomiting
	❑ Diarrhea
	❑ Abdominal pain
	❑ Stomach cramps
	❑ Choking
Respiratory:	❑ Difficulty and/or noisy breathing (Stridor)
	❑ Swelling of the tongue
	❑ Swelling or tightness in the throat
	❑ Difficulty talking or hoarse voice
	❑ Wheeze or persistent cough
Mental:	❑ Dizziness
	❑ Loss of consciousness and/or collapse
	❑ Sense of doom
	❑ Sense of fear
Taste:	❑ Metallic taste in mouth

THE "ARE YOU AT RISK" TEST

(This could save you or your child's life)

1. Symptoms: on the previous page tick the box if you or your child had any of those symptoms – count the number of ticks you marked

   ____

2. Causes or "triggers": tick the boxes below if any of the following happened and you believe could be related to the symptoms you have ticked:

❑ Ate something that immediately or within a couple of hours, you suspect caused the symptom(s)

❑ Stung by a bee, wasp. hornet or yellow jacket insect.

❑ Bitten by an insect.

❑ Took medication

❑ Contact with something that contained latex e.g. balloon, kitchen gloves, adhesive bandage or condom.

❑ Had an allergy injection

❑ Required medical care for any of the symptoms you have ticked above

RESULTS

If you had any of the symptoms ticked, you or your child may be at risk for anaphylaxis. The more ticks you marked, the greater is your risk.

If you ticked any one of the causes, "triggers" or events you think may be related to the symptoms ticked, then your risk is greater.

EVALUATION

You must appreciate ONLY your health care provider can definitively diagnose your risk situation and the purpose of this self test is to encourage you to see your health care provider to decide if you are definitely at – risk and need the auto injector and appropriate training.

It is also important to note that it is quite possible to have a mild or moderate allergic reaction before a full blown severe life threatening allergic anaphylactic reaction occurs later in the future. Consequently you or your child may still be a candidate for the auto injector to ensure complete safety.

SOMETHING TO THINK ABOUT

More than 50% of patients at risk for anaphylaxis do not know the cause (70% in adults), no matter how well done or exhaustive the search. This is called idiopathic anaphylaxis. This is very important to appreciate and you should not have unrealistic expectations that the cause can be found. Our medical consultant editors feel it is worth emphasizing that for these at -risk patients it is vital to always keep an automatic injector with them because of the unknown nature of the allergen.

CASES OF ANAPHYLAXIS

Case 1

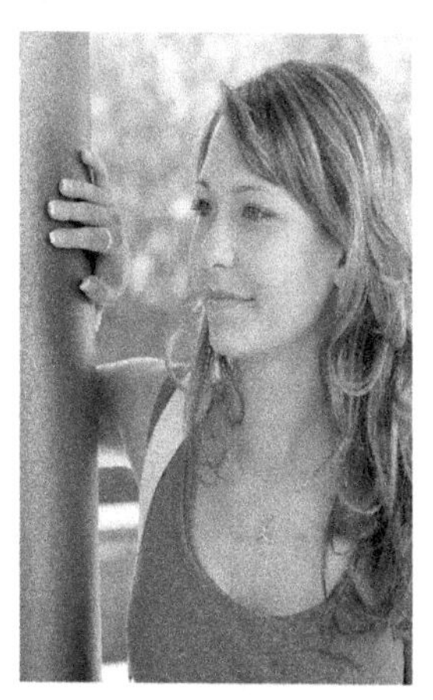

Christina: This 15 year old girl, who fairly frequently suffered from asthma attacks, but was an accomplished basket ball player and led a normal life, usually able to control the asthma attacks quickly with her puffer. She was also at risk for anaphylaxis, being allergic to nuts, but over the years had effectively avoided this allergen.

However she apparently died from the ingestion of brownies cooked and brought to her by her aunt. The aunt knew Christina was allergic to walnuts and made sure she read the ingredients on the brownie mix before preparing it, baked the mix and then drove to Christina's home with the brownies.

Later, within 5 minutes of Christina eating one of the brownies she started to have trouble breathing, she thought it was an asthma attack and rushed downstairs to the basement to find her puffer. Her friend Jack who was in the basement saw Christina inhale her medication but she was still struggling to breathe, and she then went back upstairs to the front door "to get some air", opened the door, but then collapsed. Jack immediately phoned 911. It had been less than 10 minutes since ingesting the brownie and Christina losing consciousness.

The paramedics arrived and found Christina's throat completely blocked, applied CPR, but had no success at reviving her.

When the paramedics were looking for her health card in her

purse they found a MedicAlert® bracelet, indicating she was at risk for anaphylaxis. There was no epinephrine auto injector found in the home.

In an attempt to find out what caused Christina's death, the family obtained the brownie mix box and on careful review, they discovered the brownie mix was prepared in a plant were nuts were processed.

This is obviously a tragic event but for the benefit of others it is worthwhile reviewing what went wrong:

Reading food labels: these should be read extremely carefully and you should appreciate that listing the ingredients does not provide complete safety for the at risk person. You often have to look beyond the ingredients for further "fine print" warnings or even ambiguity being a reason not to purchase.

No MedicAlert® bracelet: When paramedics and others see someone taking the trouble to wear this proactive "voice", it provides a clue to what may have taken place. It should always be worn.

No Epinephrine auto – injector: Often when people know the cause of their anaphylaxis risk and feel in control at avoiding the allergen (in Christina's case, nuts) then this can give a false sense of security.

Communication and expectations: The risk of anaphylaxis must always be communicated front and center, even though Christina had not had an anaphylaxis for a long time, it is important for family members and caregivers to be aware.

Asthma and Anaphylaxis similarities: Anaphylaxis can be confused with asthma and if there is doubt, injecting with epinephrine will not cause harm in any event.

Case 2

Tommy: This 10-year-old was up to bat when he was suddenly stung by a bee on his shoulder. He yelped with pain and brushed away the bee. Within a minute his face began to swell up, blotches or hives appeared all over his skin and he began to find it difficult to breathe.

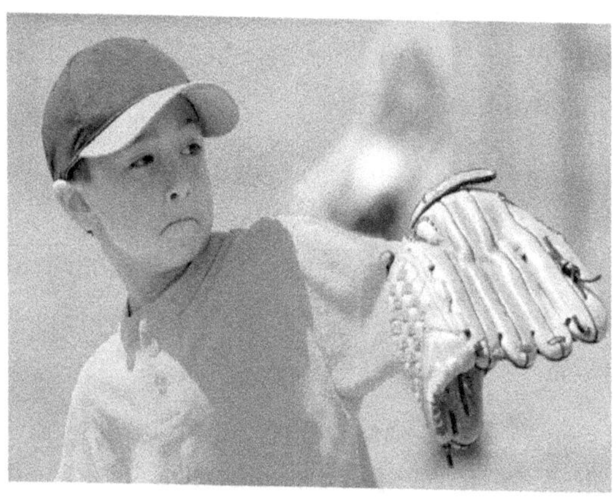

Tommy's mother was watching from the stands. She rushed down to the field and injected her son on the side of his thigh with the epinephrine auto injector and bundled him into the car. Using her cell phone, she called the emergency room of the local hospital and told them she was bringing Tommy in with a life-threatening anaphylaxis reaction.

This story has a happy ending – by next Saturday Tommy was playing in the finals, his mother standing by with her trusty auto injector, cheering from the stands.

TESTING FOR ANAPHYLAXIS

Several studies have shown that even if you have had only a mild allergic reaction to a particular food or insect bite, in time anaphylaxis may occur with a future encounter with the same allergen. Consequently you should consult with your physician on taking appropriate preventative measures.

Also, if you have had a severe but non life-threatening allergic reaction to a food or insect bite, there is a chance this can evolve at a later date to anaphylaxis. Again, you should seek a preventative plan of action for yourself or your child.

The anaphylactic condition often arises in childhood but it can occur at any age.

It requires a team effort between you and your allergist or primary care physician in order to diagnose an anaphylaxis risk to foods, medication or to insect bites or stings. Therefore, it's essential that you describe to your health care provider the symptoms you experience and what you think may be causing the symptoms. It can be helpful to record the following:

- Symptoms felt (severity, type etc.) _______________________________
- How soon symptoms developed after eating or taking a medication ____
- How long symptoms lasted after eating or taking a medication ____
- The food(s) eaten or medication taken prior to the onset of symptoms ____
- Any similar experiences you have had before _______________________

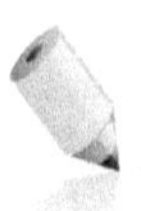

The next step is to find out objectively and scientifically what you are allergic to; this can be done by of two ways:

Allery Skin Tests

The allergy skin test can be done by placing a drop of the substance being tested on the forearm or back. The droplet is then pricked through the drop with a special needle - like instrument, allowing a tiny amount to enter the skin.

Another form of test may be necessary for insect stings and drugs. In this case a tiny amount of substance tested is injected via an extremely fine needle into the skin.

Using either test, if you are allergic to the substance, itching, redness, and sometimes swelling forms at the site within about 15 minutes.

Blood Test

A small blood sample is needed for the Radioallergosorbent test (RAST) or a CAP ELISA (enzyme linked immunosorbent assay). The sample is sent to a medical laboratory where tests are carried out to determine if you have immunoglobulin antibodies (called IgE) to these foods. The results are received back within a week or so.

There is another test called the "elimination diet" that your physician may carry out. However this can take a while as it is a sort of trial and error approach.

Your health care provider must combine the test results along with your medical history and what you have told him to make the diagnosis. Your health care provider may also give you a questionnaire to complete.

CAUSES OF ANAPHYLAXIS

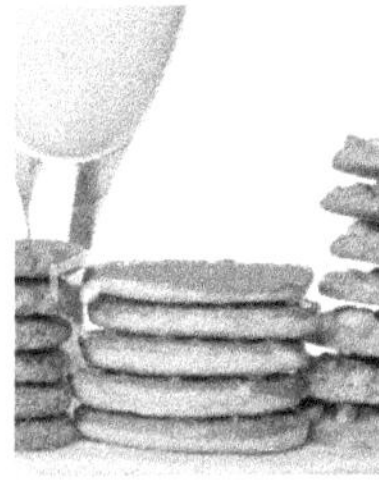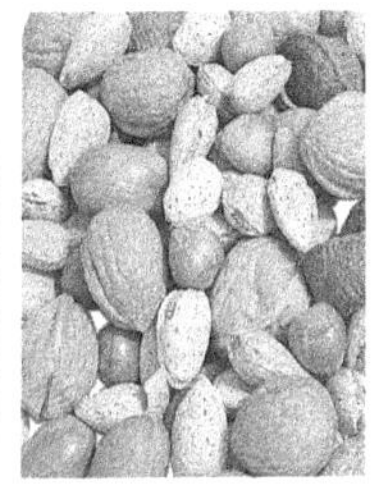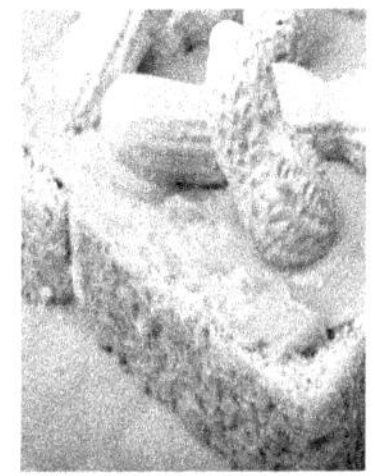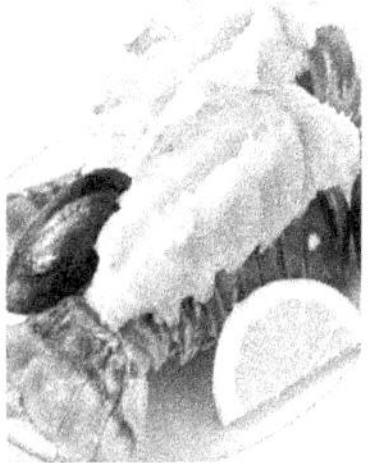

Food

The most common triggers are milk, eggs, peanuts, tree nuts (almond, Brazil nut, cashew, macadamia, hazelnut or filbert, pecan, pine nut, pistachio, walnut), sesame seeds, soy, wheat, fish and shell fish.

However, any food is capable of triggering anaphylaxis; even in small amounts food can cause a life-threatening reaction and in extremely sensitive individuals, the smell alone can trigger an attack.

Food additives such as sulfites, found in alcoholic beverages, dried fruits, vegetables, potato products, pickles and other foods can also trigger serious allergic reactions. In fact the FDA has banned sufites from fruits and vegetables,

Insect venom

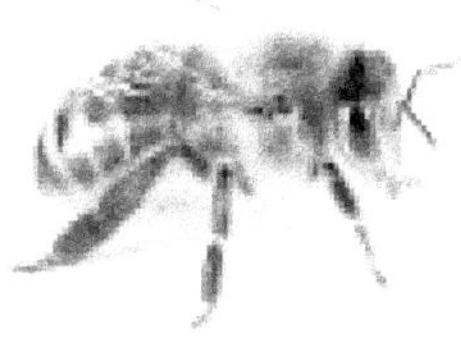

Bee, wasp, yellow jacket, hornet and fire ant stings are the most common causes of anaphylaxis.

Medication

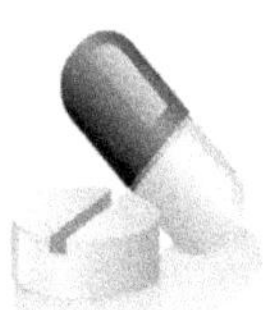

Both over the counter and prescribed medications can potentially trigger an attack. Antibiotics like penicillin are the main culprits.

Vaccines are another possibility.

Allergy shots can sometimes bring on an anaphylactic reaction. For this reason it is important to remain in the physician's office for at least 30 minutes or longer if suggested by the physician administering the injection.

Other

Latex is less common, the source can be balloons, kitchen cleaning gloves, condoms (sometimes), elastic and adhesive bandages.

Very rarely strenuous exercise can bring on an anaphylaxis.

Food allergy and food intolerance.

An adverse reaction to food can also be intolerance as opposed to an allergy. This is a completely different thing and it is worth explaining the difference.

A food allergy occurs when the body's immune system mistakenly believes that a particular food is harmful.

In order to protect the body, your immune system creates antibodies to that food, these are called the IgE (immunoglobulin E) antibodies.

Now the next time you eat that particular food, these IgE antibodies sense "danger" and signal the immune system to release massive and disproportionate amounts of chemicals and histamines which cause the unwanted allergic reactions and of course if it is severe, it can be a life threatening anaphylactic reaction.

With food intolerance, the immune system is not involved. The problem is more of a metabolic disorder where for whatever reason (perhaps a missing digestive enzyme) the digestive system finds it difficult to digest a particular food and unpleasant gastro - intestinal symptoms occur like gas, bloating and abdominal pain. These are all quite different symptoms from a food allergic reaction.

Many people go through life not knowing they have a food intolerance problem because the symptoms are often just marginal and people consider it normal for them.

There are ways of diagnosing food intolerance through a minute blood test which is quite accurate. Another alternative is to implement an elimination diet and try to pinpoint foods that are causing the problems.

WHEN IS ANAPHYLAXIS LIKELY TO OCCUR?

For both adults and children, the greatest risk of exposure is in new situations or when normal daily routines are interrupted.

Any of the following situations, where you are out of your normal routine, can provide the setting for an attack: birthday parties; camping trips; school trips; holidays; eating at restaurants, or traveling.

Young children are possibly at greatest risk to accidental exposure because they have to rely on the competence of school staff, caregivers, nannies, parents and other people who may be looking after them and who perhaps don't understand the situation or aren't trained to deal with an emergency situation.

Teenagers may be at a greater risk than young children because of the following:

- Their new-found independence, combined with inexperience;
- Peer pressure, which can relax their usual precautions;
- Reluctance to carry the auto injector medication;
- The possibility of confusing the symptoms of anaphylaxis with the onset of an asthma attack.

Previous moderate allergic reactions: Unfortunately, you and your physician must evaluate this factor – having a previous mild reaction to a food or insect <u>cannot be relied upon to predict a low risk of anaphylaxis.</u> Your physician will often recommend you carry an auto injector to be on the safe side.

MedicAlert® IDENTIFICATION

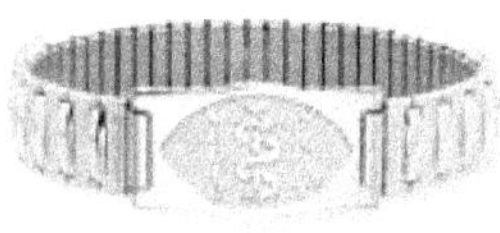 The MedicAlert® bracelet or necklace is an attractive identification shown in the illustration. It is engraved with the wearer's medical condition, membership number and the 24 hour MedicAlert® Emergency Response telephone number. This center can provide further medical information and also calls the members emergency contacts. Phoning MedicAlert® at the time of anaphylaxis can be a lifesaving action.

The enquiry phone number in US is 800 904 7629 and in Canada is 800 668 1507.

FATAL ANAPHYLACTIC FACTORS

A recent report listed several key factors that have contributed to fatal allergic reactions:

1. There was no epinephrine injected into the patient at the time of anaphylaxis.

2. Delaying the injection of epinephrine.

3. Not having a second auto injector.

4. Not dialling 911.

5. Not wearing a MedicAlert® identification bracelet or necklace

6. The failure of the anaphylactic individual to protect himself from an accidental exposure.

7. Not going to the hospital emergency clinic.

8. At-risk persons failing to acknowledge that even a tiny amount of the allergen can kill.

9. At-risk persons failing to acknowledge the seriousness of the problem, in that death can occur due to the allergic reaction.

10. Minimizing or denying the symptoms of a previous first non fatal anaphylactic reaction.

11. Failing to speak out when a reaction is first suspected.

12. Forgetting to check food labels carefully.

13. Sharing foods or utensils.

14. Obtaining food from others when the content is unknown.

15. Relying on waiters and service personnel in a restaurant instead of checking with the chef.

16. The failure of institutions to label or identify allergens to protect people from accidental exposure.

17. The failure to communicate with a babysitter, caregiver or nanny about an at-risk person and what to do in case of an emergency.

18. The failure of treatment – for example, incorrect administration of the auto injector.

19. Not empowering and training the child to communicate to people about his or her at-risk situation with anaphylaxis.

TREATMENT OF ANAPHYLAXIS

1. The epinephrine self injection or auto injection should be administered immediately at the first warning signs, such as itching and swelling of the lips or mouth, tightening of the throat or nausea, and before respiratory distress, stridor or wheezing occurs. Usually you inject in the side of the thigh slightly to the front.

2. 911 should be called or the anaphylactic patient taken to the hospital to receive immediate medical attention, even if the epinephrine has been injected and symptoms have disappeared. Symptoms may reoccur as long as eight hours after initial exposure to the allergen and more intensive treatment may be required.

3. Additional epinephrine should be available for use. A second dose should be given 5 - 10 minutes if relief has not occurred, and you have not reached a medical facility . As many as approximately 30% of anaphylactic episodes require 2 doses.

The reason for taking epinephrine (also known as adrenaline) is to assist the cardiovascular and respiratory systems by constricting blood vessels and increasing blood pressure and relaxing the chest muscles and widening narrowed airways to improve breathing.

There are no contra indications to using epinephrine for a potentially life threatening allergic reaction – immediate response is essential.

Epinephrine Auto Injectors

As a footnote to the treatment procedure using epinephrine auto-injectors, it is important to be trained and familiar with how to use auto – injectors.

There are "trainer kits" available, your health care provider can explain and there are two very useful websites for the two brands available, EpiPen˚ and Twinject˚. See website listings

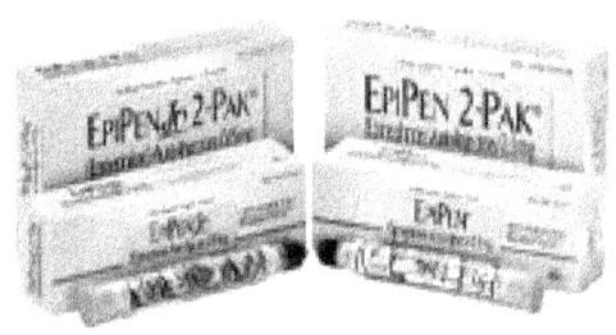
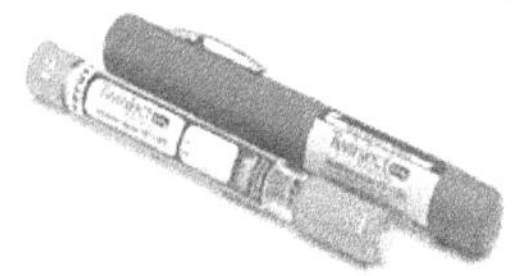

YOUR ACCESS TO AUTO - INJECTORS

Many allergists including our consultant editors give patients more than one prescription for an auto - injector. The reason being, it is understandable that patients sometimes forget to carry their auto - injector or do not want to be bothered by its inconvenience. Although it is highly recommended that you should always carry the auto - injector, the extra ones should be stored in appropriate places like at school, work, home or the car, just in case.

As a side note to the above - even if an auto injector has been stored in a car and has been subject to heat - it is believed to offer some benefit and would be harmless to administer. Also, for perhaps the teenager wearing tight jeans, and find the auto - injector bulky, there are attractive carrying cases available which can be attached to the belt.

EMERGENCY ACTION PLAN

Anaphylactic events are unpredictable so an emergency action plan is essential so that clear instructions and contact information is available. Caregivers, nannies, babysitters, relatives, spouses, friends or simply anybody in the sphere of influence should know of the emergency action plan.

The document must be easily available, a wallet card, a poster, a written document that is easily accessible and known to relevant people.

The information should include the at risk person's name , photo, what causes anaphylaxis, symptoms likely to occur, location of epinephrine auto injector, instructions on how to use the auto injector, ambulance contact details, cell phone numbers, local hospital details etc.

A sample action plan in the form of a fridge poster is shown on the next page.

This poster may be available at your physicians office or local pharmacy, if not e mail mediscript30@yahoo.ca.

Hey Babysitter, Nanny, Caregiver, Teacher or Friend

EMERGENCY ACTION PLAN

In case of a possible Severe Allergic Reaction
(called ANAPHYLAXIS)

Place child's photo here

Child's name:

Nickname:

Address:

Date of Birth:

Medic Alert #

Home phone:

Parent / guardian:

Work phone:

WARNING SYMPTOMS AND SIGNS

- ☐ Swelling (eyes, lips, face, tongue)
- ☐ Difficulty breathing
- ☐ Difficulty swallowing
- ☐ Coughing
- ☐ Choking
- ☐ Fainting
- ☐ Unconscious

- ☐ Cold, clammy, sweaty skin
- ☐ Stomach cramps and / or diarrhea
- ☐ Flushed face or body
- ☐ Change of voice
- ☐ Dizziness
- ☐ Confusion
- ☐ Vomiting

WHAT TO DO

1. **TELEPHONE 911** for emergency medical help and tell the dispatcher:

"A CHILD IS HAVING A LIFE THREATENING ANAPHYLACTIC (pronounced an - uh - fuh - lak - tik) REACTION"

2. **INJECT** with our child's emergency treatment kit.

Brand name:

Kept or stored in:

Simple instructions for use are permanently attached to the auto-injector.

OUR CHILD IS ALLERGIC TO THE FOLLOWING: PLEASE AVOID AT ALL COSTS!

☐ **Peanuts** ☐ **Tree nuts** ☐ **Milk** ☐ **All dairy** ☐ **Eggs** ☐ **Shellfish** ☐ **Fish**

Food additives (list)

Medications (list)

Insect stings (list)

Others

The overall management of anaphylaxis.

If you have a severe allergy and are at risk for anaphylaxis it is worthwhile to appreciate the official approach to medically managing you or your child's condition, as you should now have an appreciation for the critical issues, they are as follows:

- Referral to an allergist specialist.
- Identification of anaphylactic triggers.
- Education on the avoidance of exposure to the triggers. (in the case of food allergies, this may require consulting with a dietitian).
- Provision of an emergency action plan.
- Regular follow – up to an allergy specialist.

AVOIDING ANAPHYLAXIS

Avoidance of a specific food allergy or insect is the cornerstone of managing or preventing anaphylaxis.

Avoiding anaphylaxis from food

There are some facts that parents, caregivers and children should know about:

- Strict avoidance of the food allergen is the only way to prevent a reaction (there is no cure as yet).
- Even trace amounts (as small as micrograms) of a food allergen can cause anaphylaxis (remember the case of Christina).
- Most people who had an anaphylactic reaction to something they ate thought that the food was safe.
- Peanut allergies are the most common cause of anaphylaxis. Unfortunately peanuts are used as additives in many food products, further complicating the dangers.
- Peanuts are a legume and are part of the peas, beans and soy family. Technically peanuts are not actually a nut but many peanut allergic patients are also nut sensitive.
- When children become allergic to food, it is usually in the first 2 years of life, often the first time they are fed the food. After the age of 3 it is less common to become allergic to a food. Peanut sensitivity tends to persist.
- Children with asthma, especially poorly controlled asthma are at more risk from a allergic reaction to food.
- Food allergies have doubled in North America over the last 10 years.

- There is at least some good news, in that some children out grow some of their food allergies. This can occur, for example to cow's milk and eggs. Some allergies, however, more frequently persist lifelong. These, for example are those to peanuts, treenuts, and shellfish.

- Try to avoid inhaling foods to which you are allergic because this could cause wheeezing and on occassion hives / welts. For example someone allergic to shellfish should be cautious about eating in restaurants (usually Japanese restaurants) where shellfish is cooked at a large table over an open grill.

Here is a checklist of tips in avoiding food allergies:

- You must find out, with the help of your physician, which food(s) you or your child is allergic to.

- Avoidance of the food allergen can also mean making sure you or your child does not actually touch the food and making sure appropriate hand washing takes place.

- Ensure cross contamination does not take place, i.e. a utensil used in preparing your food was used with a food allergen earlier.

- Use extreme caution in restaurants, checking with the chefs (not just the waiter) that your food allergen is not included in your meal.

- Make sure your food allergen is not a hidden ingredient or additive within a meal, e.g. peanut oils used frequently in Asian cooking.

- Check food labels and make sure you understand food labels. Since January 2006 manufacturers of foods must list common food allergens on their labels. A useful website which explains how to read food labels is www.foodallergy.org, the Food Allergy & Anaphylaxis Network.

- Take lunches to work or school from home to be on the safe side as much as possible.
- Always wash your hands before eating.
- Find delicious recipes that absolutely do not contain any food allergen and possibly prepare these meals at the beginning of the week and put them in the freezer. This takes away some of the stress in planning and adapting during the week.

Avoiding Anaphylaxis risk to insects

More than 2 million North Americans are allergic to stinging insects but not all of these people are at risk for anaphylaxis. Although insect bites and stings cause thousands of trips to hospitals each year, just 50 to 150 deaths are recorded annually through anaphylaxis caused by insects. The majority of stinging insects are bees, yellow jackets, hornets, wasps and fire ants (the latter are only in the southeastern US).

There is a treatment option of "allergy shots" or insect venom immunotherapy which can protect you against future allergic reactions. You would have to discuss this with your allergist. However if you do have these allergy shots, it is important to remain in fyour physician's office for at least 20 minutes or longer so that if a reaction to the injection should occur , you can be treated promptly.

Here is a checklist of tips for avoiding stinging insects:

Preventing encounters

- ❑ Check for presence of bees, wasps and hornets, especially nesting areas and arrange for their removal.
- ❑ Never attempt to remove insect nests yourself. Always hire a professional exterminator.
- ❑ If a bee or wasp lands on you, try to gently blow it away. You should never slap or brush the insect off you or your child.
- ❑ If a bee or wasp flies into your car, simply open all the windows and it will probably fly out.
- ❑ In the event of a sting and the barbed stinger is left in the skin, never pinch the stinger. Try to flick the stinger out with a finger nail or credit card. The objective is to minimize the amount of venom injected into the skin.
- ❑ Caution children not to throw sticks or stones at insect nests or poke at them.
- ❑ Avoid the following when outside or gardening: old trees, shrubs, large rocks, woodpiles, logs, clover, heather and eaves and shutters of buildings.
- ❑ Be cautious around bird baths, pet bowls, puddles where insects prefer to feed.

Clothing prevention

- Avoid wearing loose, hanging clothes in which insects can become trapped.
- Choose clothing that covers the arms and legs when outside.
- Avoid wearing floral patterns, blue and yellow clothing or any bright colors.
- Avoid denim and corduroy, which attract insects.
- The preferred colors for clothing are white, green, tan and khaki.
- Apparently bees find black irritating and blue comforting.
- Avoid colognes, perfumes, scented lotions, soaps and hairsprays when outside.
- Always wear closed – toe shoes outdoors, avoid going out barefoot.
- Be cautious on the beach, sand can also harbor certain types of wasps.

Insect / food tips

- Always keep food covered and approach picnic areas cautiously.
- Be aware that leftover food and strong smells attracts insects.
- Avoid consuming candies, popsicles, ice cream cones and soft drinks outdoors during warm weather, Stinging insects are attracted to sweets.
- Keep the area around garbage cans as clean as possible and clean the cans with insecticide.
- Keep garbage cans covered.

CHILDREN AT – RISK FOR ANAPHYLAXIS

Parents of children with life – threatening allergies continuously walk a tightrope, trying to protect their children from exposure to even a minute amount of a common food item like peanut butter or even milk, without depriving them of a normal childhood.

Usually the child learns early in life to take their allergies seriously. The chances are that before they reach school age they have had more than one serious allergic reaction which has gotten their attention and subsequent motivation to avoid this happening again.

Over time, they learn to check food labels, have the social and communication skills to say no to certain foods and eventually will carry an auto injection of epinephrine.

With this in mind it becomes obvious that the school environment and the understanding of school staff and the children's peers becomes a critical cooperation factor in keeping safe.

Obviously it is important for the child to be well trained and empowered to manage this condition but it will make the challenges a lot easier if there is the support, knowledge and understanding from school staff. Occasionally with the challenges of the need for extreme caution combined with the usual activities of the child's age group, some children may become frightened and withdrawn, which will need addressing.

Even though a child may carry his own auto injector, it is still important to have a trained adult on hand in case of an anaphylactic reaction.

Routine is the main ally of an at – risk child in protecting young children from exposure to the allergen. When there is a field trip or a camping trip, then these are the times to take extra precautions at all levels, from auto – injectors being taken along to having special meals made prior to the trip.

Another factor to be aware of is the teasing and bullying that can happen in the child's environment when other children know someone is different or has a challenge that can be exploited in their mind, for fun.

Many cities have support groups which may be worth investigating.

TEENAGERS AT – RISK FOR ANAPHYLAXIS

Young children with life – threatening allergies are most at risk due to accidental exposure. For the parent or school staff this is a risk that can be avoided with solid preventative actions and good communications to all concerned.

However many allergists believe that teenagers, because of their new found independence, are a greater risk to fatal anaphylactic reactions.

As students reach their teen years, they become bolder, more experimental, less willing to follow the rules, and more likely to move away from familiar places and routines. Adolescent males can also perceive themselves as invincible.

Peer pressure becomes an influential factor and teenagers may not take their auto injectors because of being labeled "different" or "weird". Further they may not tell their friends of the possibility of a dangerous anaphylactic reaction and symptoms may be ignored by their friends.

A further variable is the teenager who is recently diagnosed as at risk for anaphylaxis and has grown up without this ordeal as a child and may have trouble adjusting to telling their friends and teachers of their potential problem, because perhaps of the perceived stigma.

Consequently all adults and parents involved with anaphylactic teens need to be a ware of the struggle to balance a growing need for independence with a degree of caution that is a challenge to most youth.

SCHOOL RESPONSIBILITIES

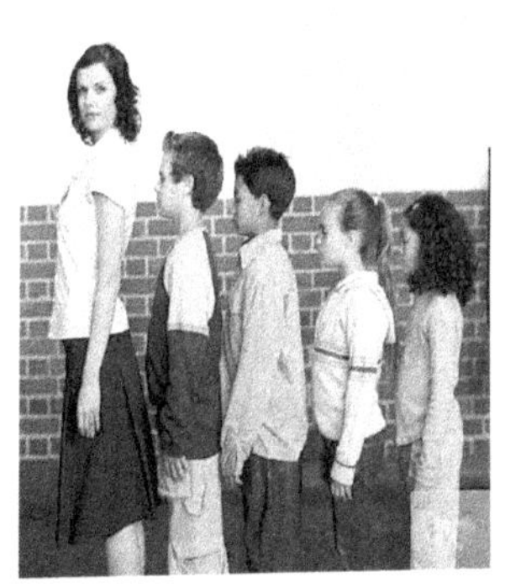

Although it is hoped the child or teenager is empowered and effective in managing his or her condition, it is helpful if the school staff are aware, understanding and trained in preventing and treating a child who is at – risk for anaphylaxis. There a lot of critical points to address but for simplicity and as a lead for taking the points to a greater depth as is needed here are some of the issues:

1. Identification of anaphylactic students to school authorities: Parents should inform the school of all the necessary information to ensure a safe environment and trained staff to ensure the safety of their child.

2. Identification of anaphylactic students to appropriate staff members: Computer listings, files, posters, symptom list, auto injector location or whatever is needed and appropriate should be used to ensure effective communication.

3. In - services for teachers and other school staff. Comprehensive in services on prevention, avoidance, what to do in an emergency as well as how to use the epinephrine auto injector should take place for full compliance for this life – threatening possible situation.

4. Sharing information with other students. With the permission of parents, the school should enlist the cooperation of other students in an appropriate manner. The use of auto injectors should also be considered as part of the awareness / training program.

5. Sharing information with parents and parent organizations
   Again with the permission of the parents, the school should
   develop a communication strategy to inform other parents of
   a student with a life threatening allergy. This can help when
   perhaps parents are sending food to the school and of course
   in many other ways.

School's approach to avoidance policies

The goal of the board's policy is to provide a safe environment for
children at – risk to anaphylaxis, but it is not possible to reduce the
risk to zero of course.

The recommendations that follow will depend upon the child's
age and maturity, and the school, parents, and student should
work together to develop and individual management plan that
includes procedures appropriate to the individual situation.

It should also be noted that precautions may vary depending on
the properties of the allergen. For example, the viscosity of peanut
butter represents challenges in terms of cross contamination and
cleaning. Milk or wheat products also pose specific difficulties in
ensuring a risk free environment.

Here are the avoidance issues which should be developed by all
concerned:

1. Providing allergen – free areas.
   This is an important issue for the lunch area, e.g. avoid eating
   in the classroom, or if that is not possible ensure an allergen
   free area within the classroom.

2. Establish a safe lunchroom and eating procedures.
   Establish non – sharing of utensils, at risk students only
   eat meals prepared at their home, increase lunch hour

supervision, placing food on waxed paper, hand washing routines established, careful choice of vending machine foods, ensuring eating surfaces properly cleaned etc.

3. Allergens hidden in school activities. Possible allergens could be in play - dough, beanbags, computer keyboards, musical instruments, asking at risk students to be involved in garbage disposal etc.

4. Field trips. Ensure the supervisor is aware of the needs of the student and is trained in the case of an emergency, an auto injector is available, ensure there is more than one dose available in case of an isolated location, permission is given for the student to participate, telephone, cell phone or other communication is available in case of an emergency

5. Substitute teachers, parent volunteers are informed. It is essential that these people are informed and trained in case of an emergency and to ensure prevention and avoidance.

6. School bus safety This environment can be dangerous for a child and the cooperation and understanding of the bus driver is needed in this situation just like the substitute teacher listed above.

7. Emergency response plan in place. Perhaps the most important factor of all because minutes can count. This plan should include knowledge of location of auto injector, administering the epinephrine injection, calling 911 immediately, if transporting to the hospital ensure you telephone ahead so they can be ready for the student, telephone parents of the child, re-administer epinephrine as needed, etc.

REASONS TO ALWAYS CALL 911

- Anaphylaxis is a life-threatening situation.

- The danger can happen within minutes – much faster than you getting to a hospital or emergency.

- The self injection of epinephrine may wear off after time.

- The anaphylactic reaction may get serious after a few hours, when you think everything is under control.

- You may need a second injection of epinephrine.

ANAPHYLAXIS SELF HELP TIPS

1. Know your anaphylaxis allergens.

2. Do everything you can to avoid anaphylaxis by research, planning, education and vigilance.

3. Ensure you carry an epinephrine auto injector kit such as EpiPen® or Twinject® and make sure you are trained on "how to use".

4. Wear a MedicAlert® bracelet.

5. Have an Emergency Action Plan see sample.

6. Communicate to family, work, school, caregivers, nannies, etc. about what to do in case of anaphylaxis and how to avoid anaphylaxis. Use posters, bookmarks, manufacturers' material and so on to keep the information front and centre.

7. Understand how to read food labels – go to www.foodallergy. org.

8. Always be on your guard when changing your daily routine like traveling, going to restaurants, visiting friends, etc.

9. Communicate with everyone around you or your child on what to do in case of an emergency anaphylaxis AND how to avoid an anaphylaxis reaction.

10. Find out about food manufacturers that specialize in allergy free foods. The list is on www.mediscript.net.

No ifs, ands or buts; when someone has an anaphylactic reaction INJECT immediately with epinephrine and CALL 911 in that order – and do both AS QUICKLY AS POSSIBLE.

USEFUL INFORMATION WEBSITES

All Allergy – internet directory of allergy organizations and resources - www.allallergy.net

American Academy of Allergy, Asthma and Immunology (AAAAI) www.aaaai.org

American College of Allergy, Asthma and Immunology (ACAAI) www.allergy.mcg.org

Allergy / Asthma Information Association (AAIA) - www.aaia.ca

Medic Alert USA www.medicalert.org
Medic Alert CANADA www.medicalert.ca

The food allergy and anaphylaxis network - www.foodallergy.org

The food allergy initiative - www.foodallergyinitiative.org

Twinject Epinephrine auto injector -
USA www.twinject.org
CANADA www.twinject.ca

EpiPen auto injector -
USA www.epipen.com
CANADA www.epipen.ca

Be Safe Program - acaai.org/member/be_safe_home.html

Anaphylaxis resources - www.aaaai.org/members/reources/
anaphlaxis_toolkit/